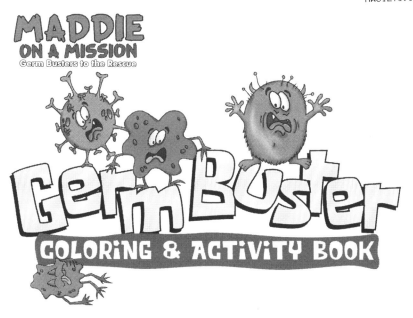

This coloring and activity book
belongs to:

_____

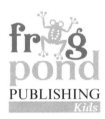
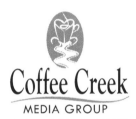

MADDIE ON A MISSION: GERM BUSTER Coloring and Activity Book
PUBLISHED BY FROG POND PUBLISHING
P.O. Box 452721
Garland, TX 75045-2721
Paperback ISBN-13: 978-1-7368929-8-5
          ISBN-10: 1-7368929-8-3

Published in the United States by Coffee Creek Media Group

MADDIE ON A MISSION NOTES

After you have read **"Maddie on a Mission,"** fill in the blanks using the words below.

LIGHT SWITCHES	SORE THROAT	SOAP	WATER
SICK	VIRUS	DOORKNOBS	PHONES
COUNTER TOPS	20 SECONDS	COLD	HEALTHY

A _____ is a tiny germ that can pass from person to person, and can

make us _____. Sick like when you get a _____, or a _____

_____.

To stay _____ and strong wash your hands with _____ and

_____ for at least _____.

To protect yourself from germs, clean things you touch often like _____,

_____ _____, _____ _____,

desks, and _____.

When you are sick, stay home and rest.

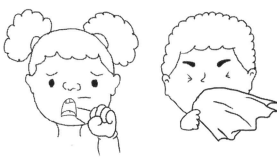

PESKY GERMS!

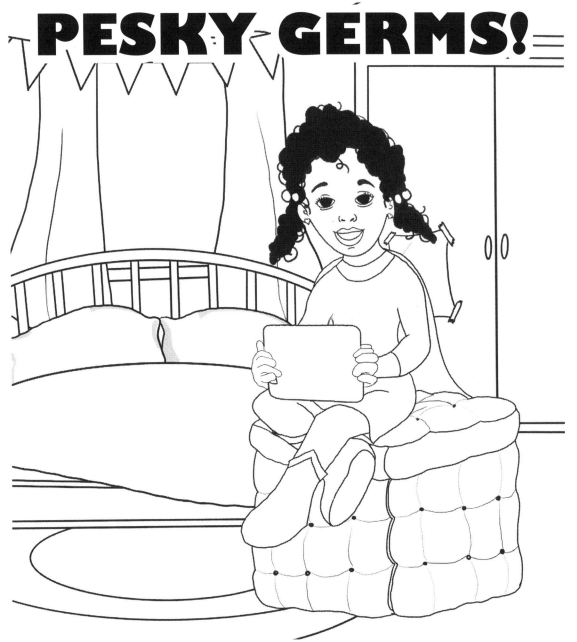

**Write ways you can keep your room germ free.
Then color the picture.**

_____   _____

_____   _____

_____   _____

   www.CoffeeCreekMediaGroup.com

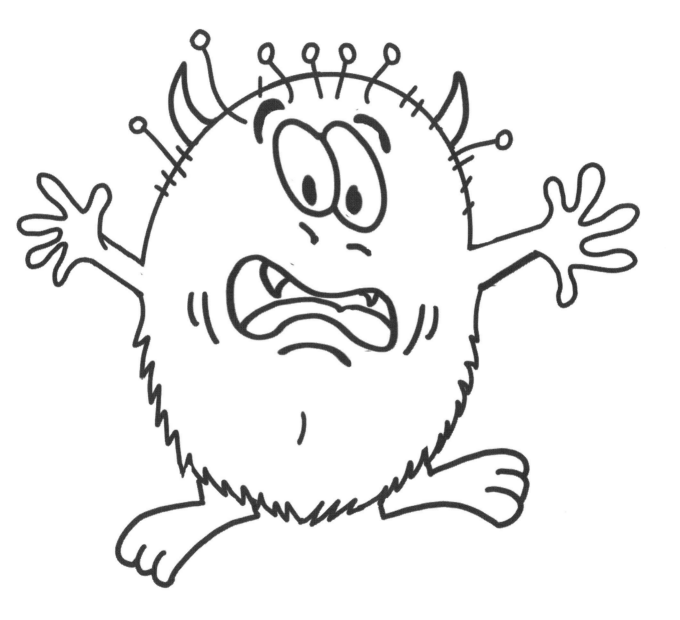

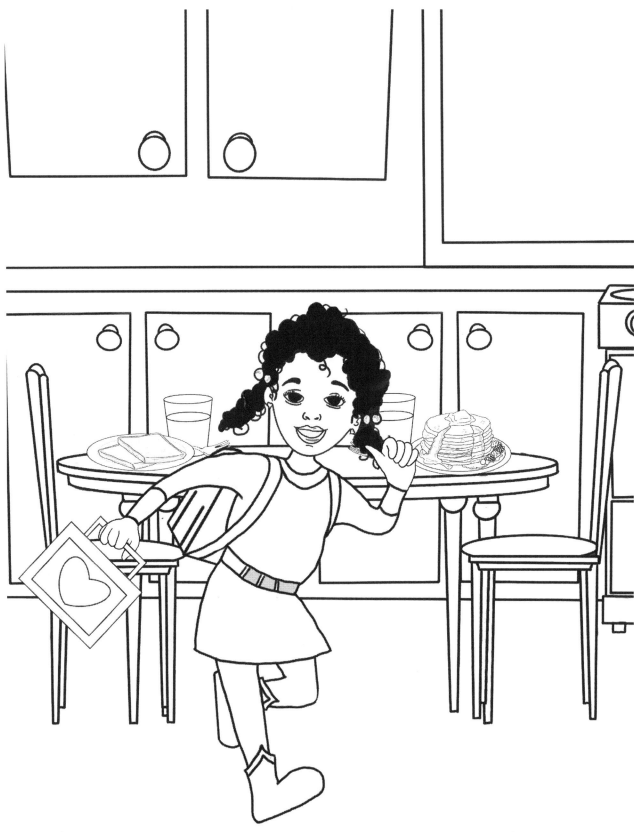

CLEAN HANDS
WORD SCRAMBLE

Unscramble the words below. Try not to use the hints.

	Hint:	Answer:
YIGHNEE	It means keeping yourself and things clean to stay healthy.	_____
RTEABIAC	Tiny organisms that can make you sick.	_____
EHATRL	It foams up when you rub it while washing hands.	_____
INRES	The last step after washing your hands.	_____
BCURS	To rub something vigorously while cleaning.	_____
SHAW	The action of cleaning your hands.	_____
NCEAL	Not dirty or messy.	_____

Name: _____

I promise to wash my hands often and keep them clean.

Be a hand-washing
Superhero!

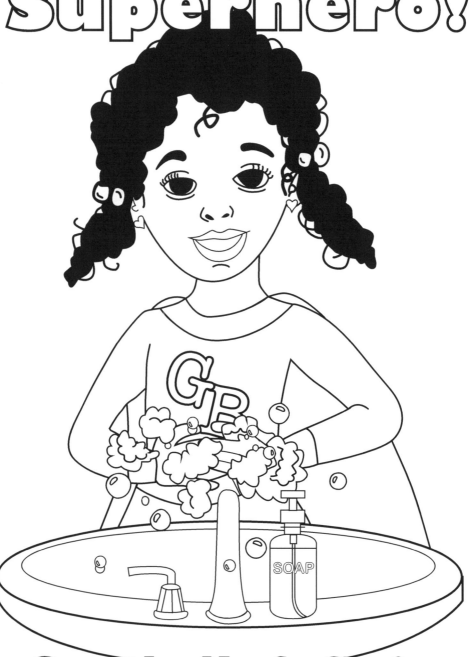

Germs Are Not for Sharing.
Please Wash Your Hands.

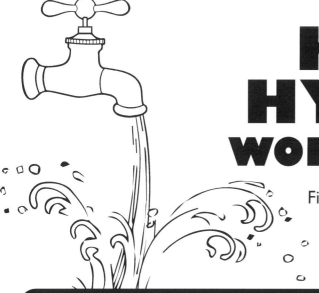

HAND HYGIENE WORD SEARCH

Find and circle the ten words in the puzzle below.

```
L D S H C B Z K C W P R R G U V O I
P A A Y U L A S E M D F X K F K S G
Q S N G Y O E B G T J G M Y Z Q C T
W D I I J N O A O N E A E U N P R X
A D T E L O B C N L E K R R P H U J
T I I N A G C T T L Q C I Y M J B U
C Q Z E T I E S C I O N E W S B K
R S A Q H F M R W I I N S M Q K I K
A L T Q E M O I P V R F E T C Z N H
J E I D R P D A U U Z C X S Y S G Y
Z A O B M J V N S W F K W L S S G K
B Z N J I S O A P B P Q N N N L Z H
```

Words are hidden → ↓ and ↘ .

BACTERIA	LATHER	SOAP
CLEANLINESS	RINSE	WATER
GERMS	SANITIZATION	
HYGIENE	SCRUBBING	

www.CoffeeCreekMediaGroup.com

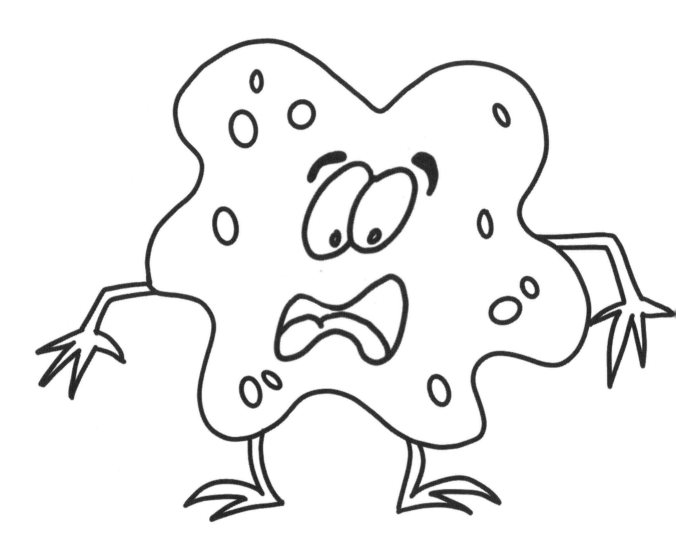

COUNT THE GERMS

Color the germs in each row based on the color listed.
Then count each and write the correct number of each type.

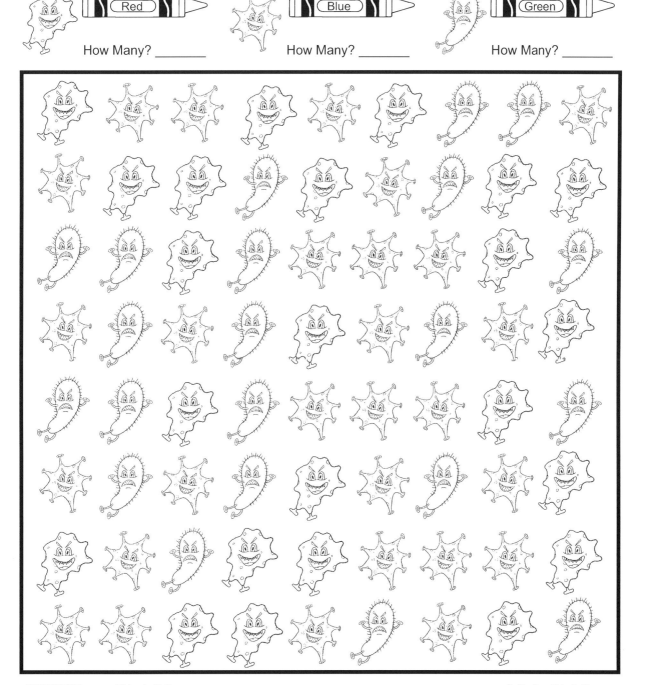

Red   How Many? _____

Blue   How Many? _____

Green   How Many? _____

GERM SEARCH

Circle each of the things where germs can live.
Color each of the things that help get rid of germs.

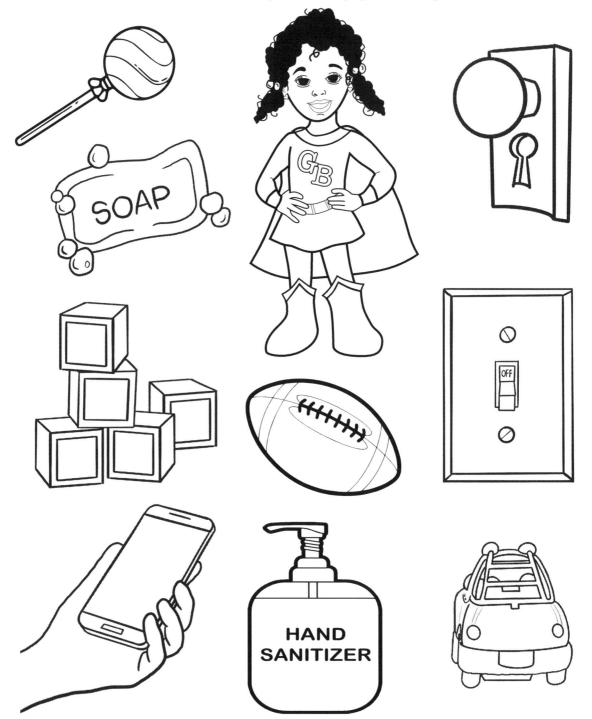

GERM BUSTER
TO THE RESCUE

Maddie is on a mission to stop the spread of germs, but she is missing her cape.
Draw Maddie's cape, then color the picture.

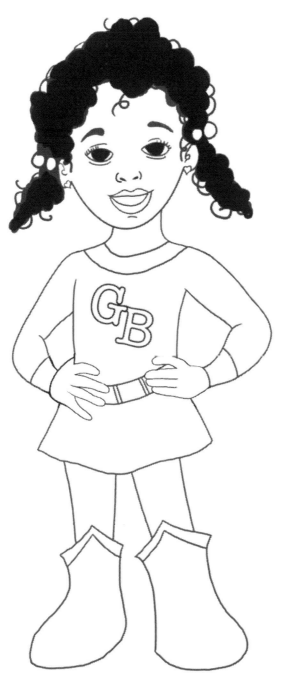

Ewww!

Draw a picture of a germ in all the sneaky spots where germs can hide on your hands!

FINGER NAILS

FINGER TIPS

THUMB

BETWEEN FINGERS

PALM

BACK OF HAND

WRIST

Time to clean your hands:
Front and back, make it grand!
Don't forget those nails down low,
And your wrists, give them a go!
Between fingers, get them clean,
Count to 20, that's the routine!

Microbiologist

I study germs.

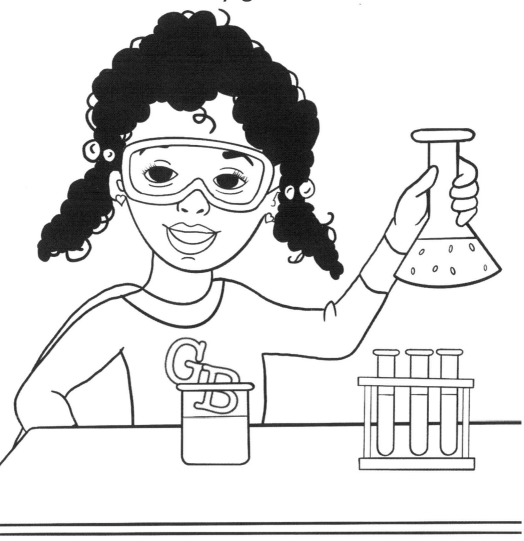

A microbiologist is a scientist who studies germs. The more we understand about germs, the better we are able to protect ourselves. Germs are so small that you need a microscope to see them!

www.CoffeeCreekMediaGroup.com

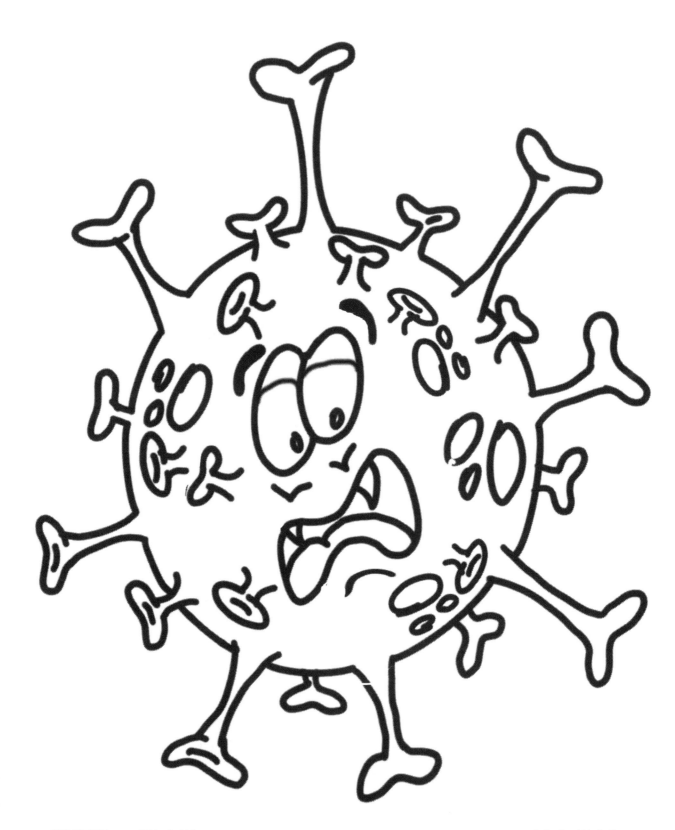

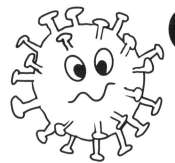

GERM BUSTERS IN ACTION!
WORD SEARCH

Find and circle the ten words in the puzzle below.

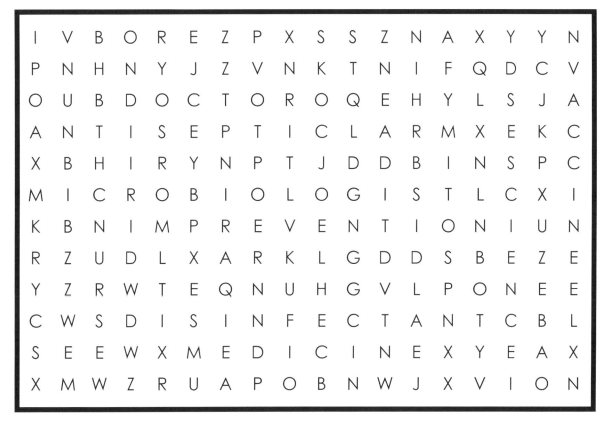

```
I  V  B  O  R  E  Z  P  X  S  S  Z  N  A  X  Y  Y  N
P  N  H  N  Y  J  Z  V  N  K  T  N  I  F  Q  D  C  V
O  U  B  D  O  C  T  O  R  O  Q  E  H  Y  L  S  J  A
A  N  T  I  S  E  P  T  I  C  L  A  R  M  X  E  K  C
X  B  H  I  R  Y  N  P  T  J  D  D  B  I  N  S  P  C
M  I  C  R  O  B  I  O  L  O  G  I  S  T  L  C  X  I
K  B  N  I  M  P  R  E  V  E  N  T  I  O  N  I  U  N
R  Z  U  D  L  X  A  R  K  L  G  D  D  S  B  E  Z  E
Y  Z  R  W  T  E  Q  N  U  H  G  V  L  P  O  N  E  E
C  W  S  D  I  S  I  N  F  E  C  T  A  N  T  C  B  L
S  E  E  W  X  M  E  D  I  C  I  N  E  X  Y  E  A  X
X  M  W  Z  R  U  A  P  O  B  N  W  J  X  V  I  O  N
```

Find the following words in the puzzle.
Words are hidden → ↓ and ↘ .

ANTISEPTIC   MICROBIOLOGIST   STERILIZE
DISINFECTANT   NURSE   VACCINE
DOCTOR   PREVENTION
MEDICINE   SCIENCE

Let's Draw!

If you were a Germ Buster, what would you look like?

Doctor

Healthy Body Exam

A*

hair — forehead
eye — ear
nose — teeth
shoulder — neck — mouth
elbow — chest
arm — stomach
finger — hand
leg
knee
ankle
foot

Doctors understand how our bodies work, and
help us get healthy again when we are sick!

Germ Buster to the Rescue

With disinfectant in hand, Maddie is ready to help fight the spread of germs! But which path is the right one?

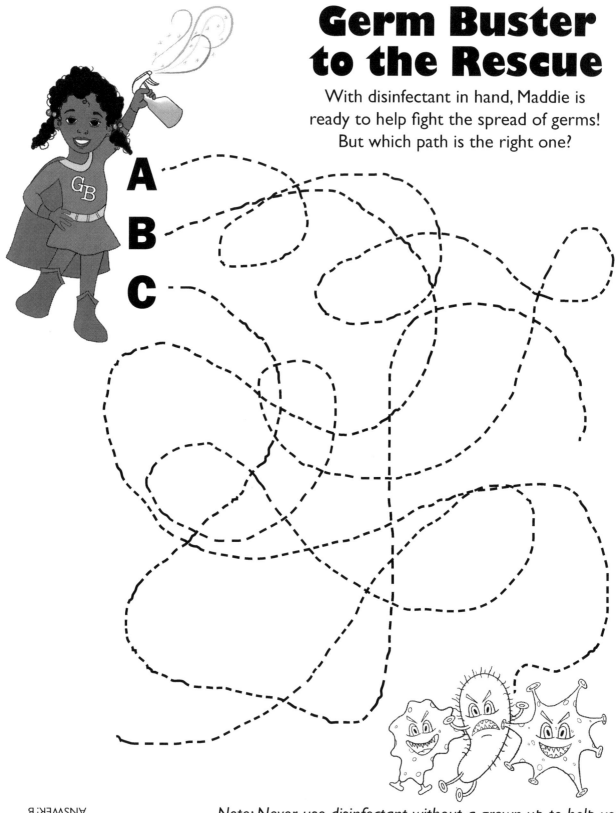

Note: Never use disinfectant without a grown-up to help you.

A Plan for Healthy Living

What foods can you eat to grow healthy and strong?

_____

_____

_____

_____

_____

What do you like to do for exercise? *(Exercise is anything that gets your body moving, like dancing, playing tag, or a sport.)*

_____

_____

_____

_____

What else can you do to stay healthy and be your best self?

_____

_____

_____

_____

_____

DOT-TO-DOT

Connect the dots 1 - 21.
Then color the germ.

Path to Recovery

Which path leads Maddie to the doctor?

START

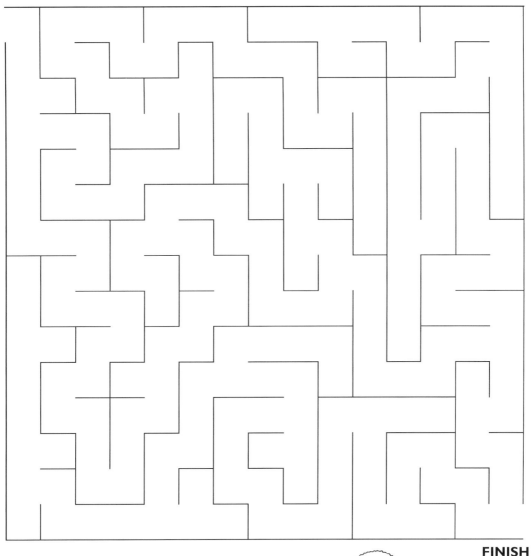

FINISH

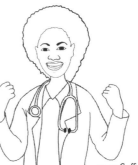

Doctors understand how our bodies work, and help us get healthy again when we are sick!

www.CoffeeCreekMediaGroup.com

Become A Germ Buster!

Let's do our part and stop the spread of germs!

Clean things that you touch often.

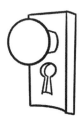 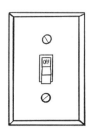 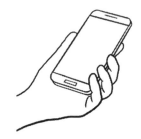

Stay home if you are sick.

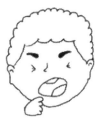 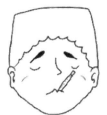 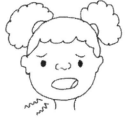

Wash your hands.

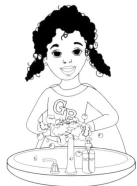

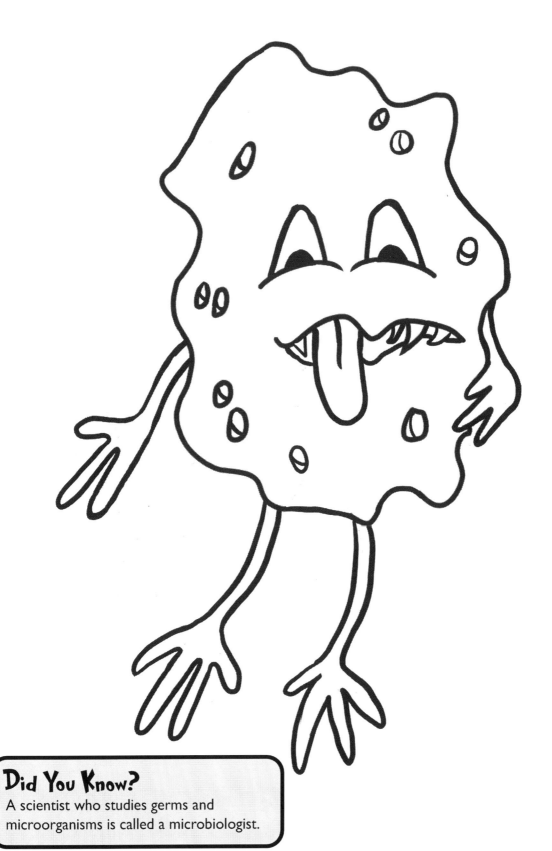

You may also like some of my other books...

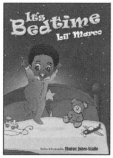 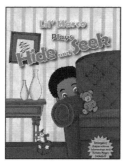 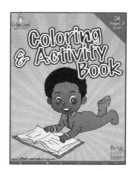 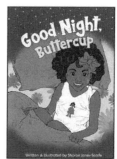 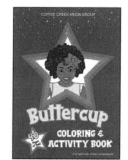

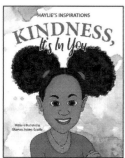 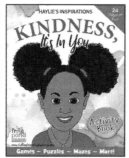 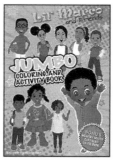 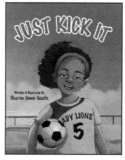 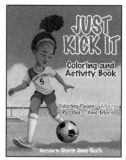

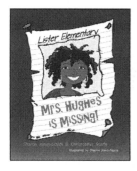 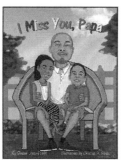 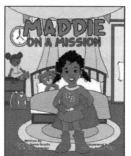 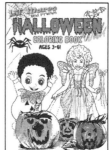 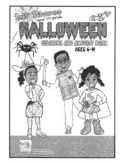

Visit my website now at www.coffeecreekmediagroup.com
or email contact@coffeecreekmediagroup.com

Follow us online

CoffeeCreekMediaGroup

SCAN ME

Available on Amazon.com

Thank you for buying my books!

GERM BUSTER BADGE

Congratulations! You have completed the activities in this book and are hereby deputized!

Color the badges below. Ask an adult to help, and carefully cut along the dotted lines.

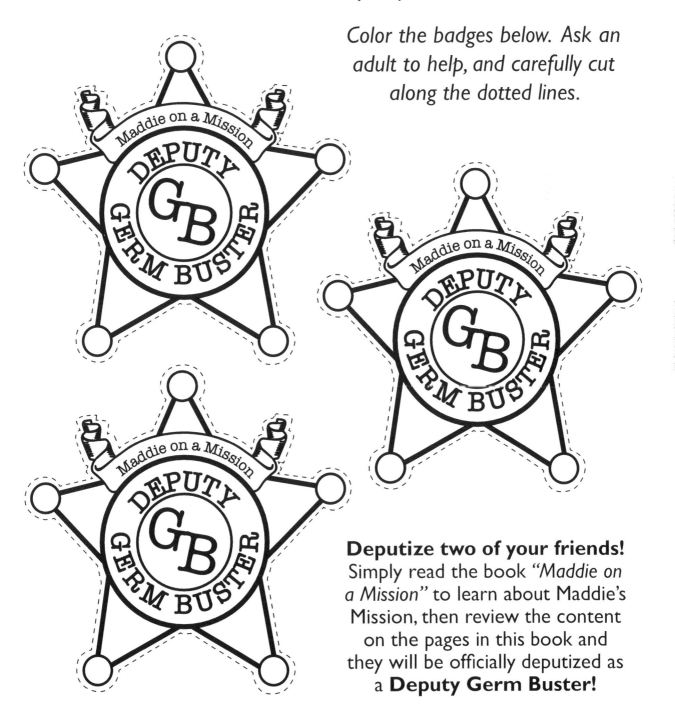

Deputize two of your friends! Simply read the book *"Maddie on a Mission"* to learn about Maddie's Mission, then review the content on the pages in this book and they will be officially deputized as a **Deputy Germ Buster!**